Thank you for purchasing our book. We hope that you find it useful in your journey to beautiful skin. Please take a moment and review this book for us. We'd love to hear your thoughts. Thank you!

Talking Gurus

Talkinggurus.com

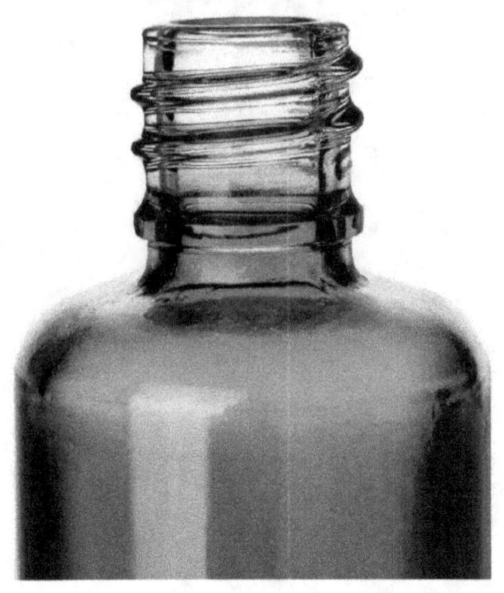
Make your own
perfect
Facial Oil

Beauty is when you can appreciate yourself. When you love yourself, that's when you're most beautiful.

Zoe Kravitz

Table of Contents

Contents

Introduction

Welcome to the wonderful world of facial oils. The intention of this book is to educate, inspire, and provide a path to creating your own perfect facial oils to address your skin care concerns. Trying to learn about facial oils can be a daunting task and it shouldn't be. There are certainly a few technical terms to be sure. However, the fun begins as you become familiar with the various properties of the different oils. For this reason, we will limit some of the excessive scientific language and focus more on the practical application of the knowledge.

Being proactive and creating your own facial oils can be an extremely rewarding endeavor. In this book we present all the information you need while avoiding hyperbole that can lead to unrealistic expectation. We have provided chapters outlining with the benefits of each oil and clarifying myths. Our first-hand knowledge and experience working with these oils is referenced throughout. Most importantly, we have provided verifiable, reputable, and independently sourced research studies to substantiate claims made about all the oils in this book. Links to these sources can be found in the *Bibliography* at the end of the book in case you want to dive deeper into the research.

Because we have been in the business of making these and other cosmetic products for companies large and small for over 20 years, it was a pleasure to create this book for you. *Make Your Own Perfect Facial Oil* is designed to provide the most essential information in the easiest format for all experience levels. You will note that therapeutic formulas are most often composed of unique blends of facial oils to address specific concerns. Bringing these oils together is known as compounding. While this book does not cover the science of compound formulating, we use the basic tenets in the chapters dealing with formulating. By the end of this book, you will have a good working knowledge of facial oils and an ingredient list of the most therapeutic oils used to make them. You should have everything you need to create your own perfect facial oils.

Chapter 1

Facial Oil Benefits And Properties

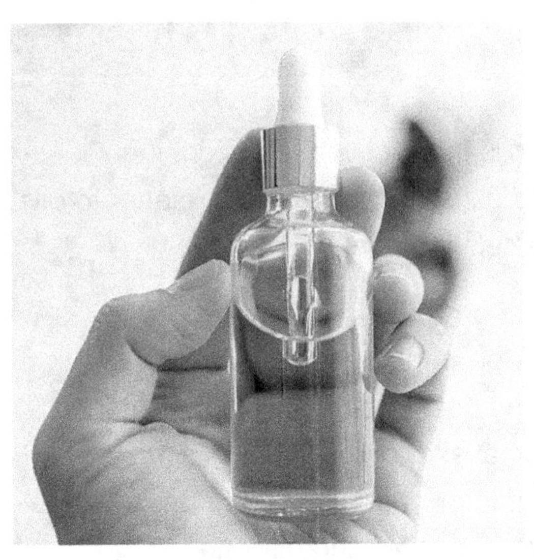

Chapter 1
Facial Oil Benefits and Properties

Understanding Your Skin

To understand how oils interact with the skin, it is helpful to understand skin functioning as it relates to oils and hydration at the cellular level.

The skin is the largest organ in the body. An entire medical specialty of dermatology is devoted to it. Estheticians and some cosmetologists specialize in the care of mostly facial skin care. There is a substantial amount of information available on the functioning of the skin, specific skin disorders, treatments, etc. For our purposes, there are basics that you need to know before crafting your own facial oils.

Skin is made up of three layers – the epidermis, the dermis, and the subcutaneous tissue. The epidermis is the outer layer that we can see. The dermis is the middle layer of skin that contains connective tissue, blood vessels, oil and sweat glands, hair follicles and nerves endings.

The subcutaneous tissue is a fatty layer within the skin that controls the amount of hydration or water in the skin, and it is hydration that gives skin elasticity, avoids wrinkles, prevents oiliness and gives skin an even tone and a youthful, healthy glow.

Lipids, also known as fats or oils, are a natural part of and play a key role in the structure of the skin. Oils keep water inside the layers of skin where it is needed to prevent dryness. This protection is provided by the outermost layer of the epidermis, called the *stratum corneum*, consisting of cells rich in keratin (corneocytes). This outer layer of the epidermis is embedded in a fatty layer made mostly of cholesterol, ceramides (a combination of fatty acids with an amino acid), and free fatty acids. Free fatty acids, as opposed to esterified fatty acids, are free to move to wherever they are needed. The lipids that make up this fatty layer are formed within a deeper layer of the skin then move to areas throughout the skin where needed. The fatty layers are organized and distributed strategically throughout the skin to ensure the skin has a barrier function. The barrier keeps the skin waterproof from the outside while also keeping water inside. If the barrier function of the skin is disrupted there is an increase in transepidermal water loss (TEWL). The result is a decrease in water content of the skin which we define as dry skin.

Practically speaking, you should know that the fat inside the skin cells.

1.) Provides a protective barrier to keep bad stuff out.
2.) Moves around within the layers of the skin to keep moisture in
3.) Has different functions depending on the type of fat or lipid.
4.) When disrupted, damaged, or lacking, leads to skin problems.

The skin relies on the fats/oils within to maintain a healthy barrier and prevent moisture loss. In a perfect world, there would be no need for facial oils. There would be no skin issues related to aging, environmental, or genetic factors. The skin would manufacture everything it needs as does the skin of healthy babies. Fortunately, we have the tools and wisdom of nature to heal, treat, maintain, and optimize the skin we have.

In the past, it was thought that oils were bad for the face and caused acne or blocked pores. But research has shown that facial oils are extremely beneficial for the skin. They can moisturize skin that may not have been helped with creams alone. They can decrease the appearance of wrinkles, protect against dry skin, and provide numerous benefits which we will discuss in this chapter.

Not all oils are the same. It is important to remember that not every type of oil is beneficial for the face. While specific oils have the ability to beautify and enhance, other oils can indeed produce clogged pores and irritation. Further, the cultivation, harvesting, and extraction methods used in obtaining facial oils may vary greatly. The best facial oils are pure, derived from reputable sources, maintained in optimal conditions, and provide consistent results.

General benefits of pure facial oils:

1. They absorb well into the skin.

Of all the benefits of facial oils, this one is the most important. Without good absorption, none of the other properties are available. Pure facial oils are lipophilic or "fat loving". That means they will pass through the outer layers to the inner fatty layers of the skin. Facial oils bring all their benefits and therapeutic properties directly where they are needed.

2. They provide anti-inflammatory support.

Specific oils can provide calming effects to skin by decreasing inflammation, itching, and providing protection against the consequences of irritated skin. These oils can not only calm down certain rashes, but they can also help relieve itchiness.

3. They protect against pollutants.

We can absorb toxins from air pollution through our skin. Whether it's big city fumes or small-town pollutants, these toxins can harm our skin. Facial oils, unlike moisturizers, provide a protective barrier against air pollutants. Many facial oils are potent antioxidants and can protect against free radical damage as well.

4. They can decrease the appearance of wrinkles and make pores appear smaller.

By increasing the ability of the skin to lock in moisture, skin cells are less dehydrated and saggy. Added moisture causes pores to appear smaller. Hydration also decreases the appearance of fine lines and makes wrinkles appear less pronounced. Pure facial oils accomplish this because they absorb so well into the skin. Once the oils are absorbed, they provide a protective barrier that serves to prevent the moisture in the skin from evaporating easily.

5. They are rejuvenating to the skin and provide a radiant glow.

"In with the good and out with the bad" is a classic motto for health. For any cells to rejuvenate, they must get rid of the bad things like toxins and natural and environmental debris. Cells must also bring in the good things, like nutrients, peptides, emollients, and hydration. Only a good blend of pure facial oils can accomplish all of this. There is no single oil that brings the good stuff in while simultaneously taking the bad stuff out effectively. Specific, time-tested combinations of pure facial oils can provide essential skin rejuvenation for a naturally healthy complexion.

Individual properties of each oil are discussed in Chapter 4 and a chart of oils with similar properties can be found in Chapter 5.

6.They help makeup apply more smoothly and evenly.

Applying liquid foundation or powders to dehydrated skin is never a good look. Moisture craved skin will suck every drop of oil or moisture from your makeup. The result will be an uneven application that becomes more uneven as the skin continues to soak up what it can throughout the day. Primers made from silicone only cover over the problem. Pure facial oils solve the problem. Providing the perfect vehicle to penetrate, "lubricate," then seal in moisture, pure facial oils give your skin a consistently smooth base for any liquid, cream, or powder makeup you want to apply.

Chapter 2

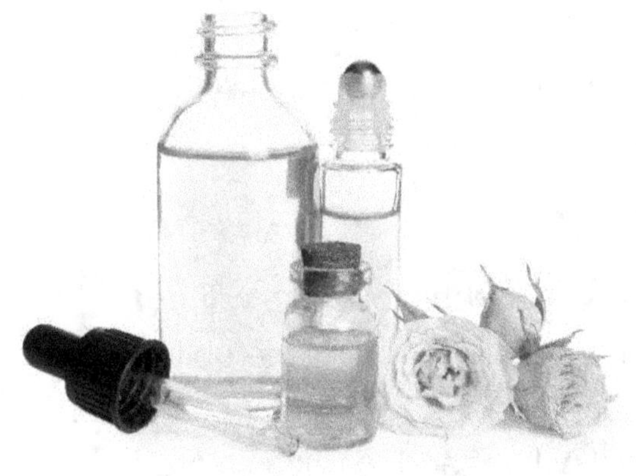

Top 6 Myths

about

Facial Oils

Not all oils are created equal and therefore not all oils should be used on the face. Oils have different intrinsic properties and behave differently when applied to the skin. Just some oils are suitable for cooking; certain oils are better suited for the face.

While there is a lot of information available, it is important to dispel certain myths. Here you will find some of the top myths about oils.

1. *Oils clog your pores*

Certain oils are non-comedogenic oils and will **not** clog your pores. "Comedogenic" means the ability to clog pores. A comedone is clogged pore that can lead to a pimple, blackhead, whitehead, or skin colored bump. The skin, as an organ, absorbs oils and nutrients, which can eventually end up in the bloodstream. Skin also keeps large molecules out because intact skin acts as a barrier. Comedogenic oils are of a particular molecular size and density to clog pores. Non-comedogenic oils are absorbed quite easily into skin and do not stay on top of the skin to clog pores.

2. Don't use oils if you have oily skin

Even before we heard about the T-zone, we have been aware that some people have naturally oily skin. Genetics, diet, and lifestyle are generally given as the causes of oily skin. We know that hormones influence the oiliness of skin. We also know that aging often produces decreased oiliness and drier skin. Scientific studies show that the oiliness of skin is not related to the quantity of total lipids in the skin but rather to the ratios of unsaturated fatty acids and wax esters in the sebum. Research further indicates that oily skin is low in linoleic fatty acids. For this reason, oils containing high levels of linoleic acid tend to work well with oily skin. Oils that are higher in oleic acids, on the other hand, do not work well with oily skin.

3. Don't use oils if you have acne

Scientific studies have consistently shown that a lack of linoleic oils can cause the skin to overproduce sebum, the naturally occurring oils that can clog pores and produce acne. Reducing acne breakouts can be accomplished with consistent cleansing routines and various topical treatments. However, many acne treatment protocols leave the skin extremely dry. Excessive dryness from acne treatments has now been shown to also cause the skin to overproduce the very oils that can clog pores. Treatments that work initially can actually make the problem worse over time. A solution can be found in pure facial oils. Non-comedogenic oils are now considered an essential part of treating acne successfully.

4. Any oil can be used on the face

It bears repeating that not all oils are created equal. While synthetic oils may soothe the skin when applied, these silicones, mineral oil, and petroleum products do not absorb well into the skin. They do not provide antioxidants or other nutrients as do pure, natural facial oils. In fact, synthetics provide no hydrating effects and can leave the skin much dryer. Certain food grade oils and even a few genuine essential oils can be bad for the skin as well.

5. Oils go bad fast

Without preservatives natural and organic oils generally have a shelf life of about one year. Some oils can spoil faster, and others can last a bit longer. Keeping your oils in a cool dry place away from sunlight and moisture helps them remain stable longer. When oils go bad, they become rancid, lose their chemical properties and can develop a bad odor.

The key to preserving all the wonderful benefits of facial oils is two-fold. First, oils with Vitamin E or tocopherol properties should be included as a natural preservative to keep the oils stable for a longer period of time. The Vitamin E or tocopherol properties are beneficial for the skin as well. Second, oils with natural antioxidant qualities should always be included in facial oil formulas. Since oxidation is the chemical reaction by which oils become rancid, antioxidants naturally slowdown that process. The antioxidant properties of the facial oil are not only beneficial for the face, but for the product as well. All of the formulas included in this book include either natural preservatives, natural antioxidants, or both.

6.   *You can use essential oils in your facial oil blends*

Essential oils are plant extracts, many of which have healing properties. A vast amount of information is available on the proper use of essential oils. There are also a few essential oils that have been studied for their use in cosmetics. While it is certainly true that some essential oils can be used in facial oil blends, all of them cannot. Generally, essential oils should never be put directly on the skin. Those that may be safely used on the skin should be mixed with a carrier oil, which can be any of the plant based facial oils discussed in this book.

Chapter 3

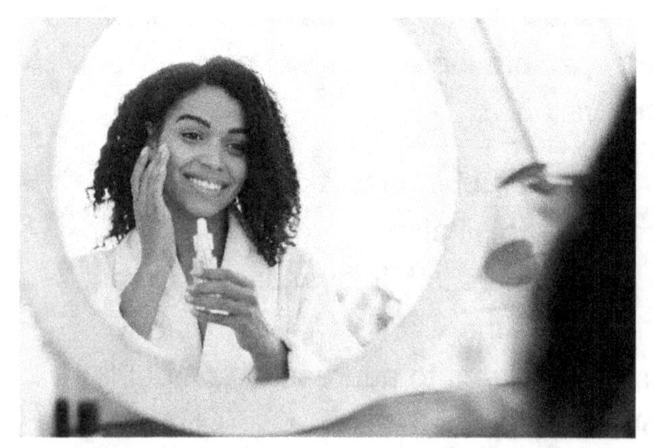

How to Use

Facial Oils

How to Apply

The first thing to know about using pure facial oils is that you don't need much. More is not always better. Begin with a drop or two in your palm and rub your hands together to warm the oil and increase its absorbability. Then pat the oil all over the face or massage the oil into the skin using upward strokes. Be careful not to get the oil into the eye which may temporarily blur the vision.

Another option is to avoid rubbing the skin by using your clean finger to tap the oil all over the face. Give your skin time to absorb the oil at its own pace. There is no need to rub it in unless there are some particularly dry or problem areas you want to address. If you get too much oil in one place, you can disperse it over the rest of the face by dabbing or patting. You can also use any excess oil on the cuticles, elbows, back of the hands, or other dry skin areas. The neck is another good place to apply oil.

When to Apply

The next thing to consider is **when** to apply the oils. First, make sure the skin is properly cleansed. If you use a toner, allow it to dry before applying oil. A facial oil will not mix with a water-based toner. The oil could block the toner from releasing its properties. Also, the toner may interfere with the oil being evenly absorbed. Since many toners have astringent properties, they can contribute to skin dryness. However, some toners contain antioxidants or other beneficial ingredients. Toners can be helpful in removing makeup that may not have been completely removed with cleansing. Consequently, it is the ingredients in the toner that dictate whether or not the toner is helpful or necessary when addressing dry skin.

Before applying facial oil you should next consider whether to apply them before, after, together with, or in lieu of your moisturizer. This is a matter of preference. Find what works best for you.

What comes next is determined by your skin type, skin care routine, and preference. Normal, average, or combination skin types have the most options. Skin routines that include acne, anti-aging, or specialized treatments will have more to consider. The order in which you apply your skin products should work for you easily and you should receive the maximum benefits from each of the products that you are using.

In general, it is recommended that facial oils be applied **after** serums, moisturizers, and specialty treatments. The rationale is to let the other products absorb into the skin to do the work they are designed to do. Then, follow with the facial oil to seal in the moisture, provide the protective barrier, and lay a smooth foundation prior to the application of any makeup. This protocol will work for most people. However, there are certain considerations which may alter this application order.

Considerations for applying facial oils:

Serums

Serums can be water-based or oil-based. They can include incredibly potent ingredient formulations or simple kitchen counter, DIY combinations. In general, it is advisable to apply facial oils **after** simple serums. The thinking is that thin, non-oily serums are considered to contain smaller molecules than facial oils, thus absorbing more readily into the skin. However, that is not always true. To deliver the benefits that they promise, serums may also contain chemical compounds, preservatives, or other poorly absorbed ingredients. If your serum contains silicones, it will not allow the proper absorption of a facial oil. Serums containing silicones boast of making skin feel smoother. That is a property of the silicone itself as it lays on the skin. Silicone does not actually change the skin in any way. Facial oils should be applied **before** serums containing silicones. A section on recognizing silicones in your products is included in this book.

Facial oils may also be applied **before** oil-based serums for convenience. These heavier serums can take a while to absorb into the skin. Applying them after a fast-absorbing pure facial oil makes sense. If absorption time is a significant consideration, the 2 may be applied together to get the benefits of both in one application.

Acne Treatments

There are many varieties of products and protocols on the market today for acne. Not all products act in the same way and what works for some may not work for others. In that regard, it is not possible to make a general statement about facial oils that will apply to every user of every product. What is considered a good rule of thumb is to apply facial oils after the other treatments have been completely absorbed and the skin is dry. Facial oils may be applied **after** a moisturizer or in lieu of a moisturizer. Try both ways and observe which method provides the best effects. It is not advisable to use an oil-based moisturizer with a facial oil in the case of acne. Neither the moisturizer nor the facial oil should contain comedogenic oils that may clog the pores.

Moisturizers

The key to a good moisturizer is the balance of oil and water. This is a product that can vary widely in consistency. It can be watery like a thin lotion, or it can be a very thick cream. Because moisturizers are not uniformly formulated, and there is no one size fits all, it is hard to make a general statement that applies to everyone. If your moisturizer is sufficiently providing you with all the hydration you need, reducing the signs of wrinkles and decreasing the appearance of pores while also giving you a nice radiant glow, that is a good moisturizer. However, if your moisturizer is not giving you all that it could, you may need a facial oil. Definitely apply facial oil **after** a thin moisturizer. That is the standard way to lock in the moisture and maximally hydrate the skin. If you are using a thick, heavy, more oil than water moisturizer, you may want to use facial oil **before** or instead of your moisturizer. The facial oil could provide you with additional benefits thus acting as a serum, or as a serum and facial oil in one. The new term that we coined for this is a "seroil".

Oily Skin

If you have oily skin, it is most important to test on your own skin. Not everyone has oily skin for the same reasons. Some people naturally produce more sebum. Other people overproduce sebum to compensate for dry skin or products that create dry skin. Even if the skin is naturally oily, it may be crying out for more of the beneficial oils. Whatever is the case, applying a small amount of facial oil can provide hydrating and nourishing benefits to the skin. When used on naturally oily skin, facial oils can often take the place of moisturizers.

SPF

The importance of SPF application cannot be overemphasized. It is particularly important to protect your skin from damage caused by the sun's UV rays. Some moisturizers provide this SPF protection and should always be applied **after** facial oils. If you are using a separate SPF product, that product should always be applied last and after the facial oil has been completely absorbed.

Silicones

Silicones are chemicals found in serums, cleansers, moisturizers, primers, facial oils, masks, and makeup. They are not dangerous and are considered safe by the FDA. There are scientific studies that show that silicones can be especially useful in sunscreens and other specialized formulations. This does not mean that repeated continual use won't lead to some unwanted problems. Silicones can create dryness, prevent the absorption of beneficial products, and be difficult to clear from the skin. What they do is lay on the skin surface like a silky film, filling in ridges and naturally occurring crevices, making the skin feel soft, even, and silky smooth. What they also do is prevent the skin from readily clearing debris, from maximally absorbing moisture from the air, and absorbing nutrients that may be applied to the skin. Silicones create a semi-permeable barrier that can make the skin feel like it's difficult to "breathe" or like it has a protective coating.

Products with silicones claim the benefits of moisturizing, hydrating, and smoothing without improving the skin itself. Once the silicone is removed, and this is not always easily accomplished, the skin is unchanged and can become duller or dehydrated with continual use. Silicones are much cheaper and last longer than naturally occurring oils and other nutrients. They are recognized by the "cone" at the end of their names. They are also known as "conols," "silanes," and "siloxanes." Ingredients composed of silicones can be known as acrylamides, acrylates, carbomers, polymers, copolymers, polybutenes, and the like. The most important thing to note is that silicones prevent the beneficial effects of facial oils by preventing their absorption. Check the ingredient label on all of your facial care products. If silicones are listed in the ingredients, know that they will prevent the absorption of the beneficial aspects of pure facial oils. These products should only be applied **after** facial oils.

Chapter 4

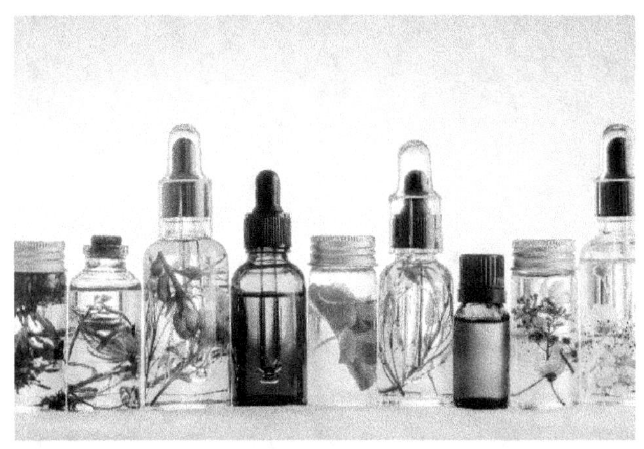

The 15 Most Powerful

Facial Oils

Many guides characterize individual oils as being good for one condition or another. This is only a small part of the picture. The truth is that botanical oils are chemically diverse. Their mode of action and how well they perform depends on the quantities and proportions of their individual chemical components. No matter the composition or ratio of components, blending oils together takes their use to another level. They are at their best when sharing their combined and synergistic effects.

While you will certainly notice the benefits from the intrinsic properties of non-comedogenic oils - moisturizing, hydrating, and barrier protection, other properties may not be as readily apparent. Antioxidant, cellular rejuvenation, and many other benefits take place beneath the surface of your skin. These benefits happen over time, but it is time well spent. Longer term use provides longer term results.

The degree to which beneficial properties manifest is often a function of how the oils are harvested, prepared, processed, and stored, as well as where the plant sources were originally grown and nurtured. Although prices vary greatly, in general, ethically sourced, and carefully harvested ingredients are not cheap. This is not to say that only expensive products are useful. In general, the rarer the ingredient is, the more expensive it is. The more widely available the oil is, the lower the price.

With this foundation of information, you can now appreciate the beauty in the science of beauty. Nature has given us our medicine. In this chapter, we have chosen the 15 most powerful facial oils readily available today. Not only do they deliver results, but all of them are quite versatile. Each of these oils will meet and/or exceed your expectations with consistent use.

Argan Oil

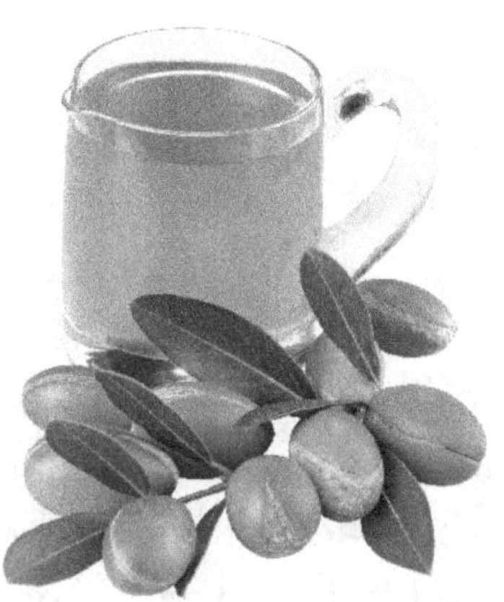

Grown only in the south-west of Morocco, the argan tree *(Argania spinosa)* is rare. The region where argan oil can grow is limited and the supply worldwide is relatively small. As a result, authentic argan oil is expensive and there have been several attempts to defraud the global marketplace with imposters.

The fruit of the argan tree is fleshy and green like an olive. It has a nut inside with an extremely hard shell. Inside the shell are one to three almond shaped kernels. Argan oil has an unusually high concentration of vitamins E and A along with other important nutrients. The oil is edible and has a high unsaturated fatty acid content, about 80% in the form of oleic and linoleic acids. Several studies have revealed many beneficial qualities of the oil making it extremely popular in the cosmetic industry. Argan oil is particularly useful in providing lubrication and cellular support for aging skin. It significantly increases the elasticity of skin, providing anti-aging effects. It also decreases transepidermal water loss and increases water content of the epidermis. Daily application of argan oil improves skin hydration by restoring the barrier function and maintaining the capacity of the skin to retain water. Twice daily application of argan oil reduces the amount of sebum and therefore naturally reduces oiliness of the skin. It also has good antioxidant properties and reduces free radical damage.

Baobab Oil

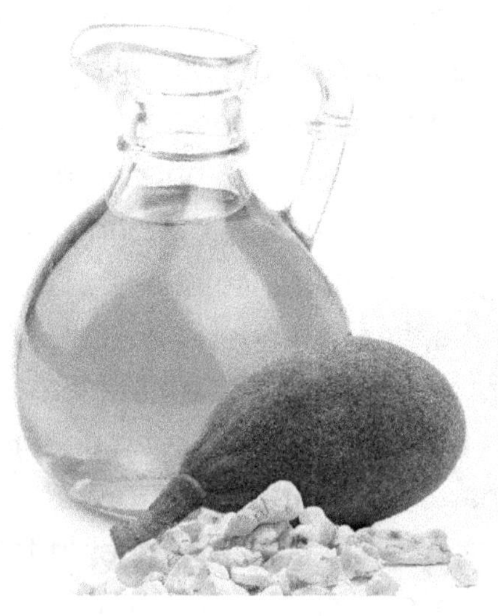

Also known as the monkey bread, the upside-down, or the tree of life, the baobab tree is regarded as the largest succulent plant in the world. The large egg-shaped fruit capsule contains numerous seeds from which the oil is extracted. Baobab, *Adansonia digitata,* fruit oil is rich in omega 3, 6, and 9 fatty acids. About 33% of the seed content is oil with oleic and linoleic acids as the primary components. Baobab oil is also high in vitamins A, C, D, E, F, and K. Vitamins A and 'F' are polyunsaturated fatty acids directly implicated in cellular renewal and rejuvenation. The unique ratio of saturated and unsaturated fatty acids is thought to contribute to the powerful effectiveness of this oil. The beneficial properties are exceptional for improving the function of the sebaceous glands and preventing comedo-acne formation. The oil absorbs quickly and is efficacious for many sensitive, oily, and problematic skin types. Baobab oil softens the skin, restoring moisture, and reducing the appearance of scars, fine lines, wrinkles, dark spots, UV damage, and stretch marks. It has significant antioxidant and anti-aging properties. It increases elasticity and collagen under the skin to help repair damaged skin. Its soothing properties are also helpful in eczema, psoriasis, and other irritable skin conditions.

Black Cumin Seed Oil

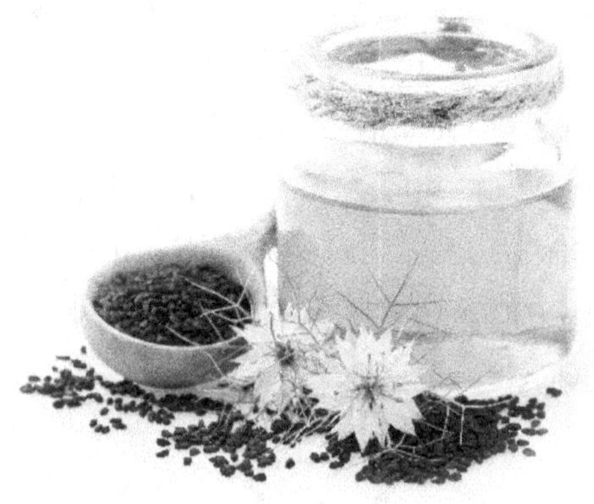

Black seed (*Nigella sativa),* also known as black cumin seed, comes from the fruit of a shrub grown in North Africa, Southern Europe, and Southwest Asia. Black Cumin Seed oil contains a substantial amount of vitamins, minerals, and omega fatty acids. Over 60% of the fatty acids are linoleic. It is nutrient dense with vitamins A, B, and C, copper, zinc, and selenium along with other skin loving nutrients. These include thymoquinone, thymol and other active phenols. Extracts of these nutrients are used in the treatment of vitiligo. Black cumin seed oil provides exceptional anti-inflammatory, antioxidant, anti-fungal, anti-parasitic, and anti-bacterial effects. It is particularly useful for treating acne, eczema, psoriasis, blisters, and many dry skin conditions. It hydrates, soothes, smoothes, and nourishes the skin. It is widely used to promote skin reparation and regeneration and provides rejuvenating and revitalizing effects. Its antioxidant activity promotes the elimination of harmful free radicals. Thus, it diminishes the appearance of fine lines, dark spots, wrinkles, and other blemishes. The anti-inflammatory properties soothe the skin and facilitate healing. In addition to all these properties, black cumin seed oil has anti-neoplastic, anti-tumor, anti-cancer activity as an extra important benefit.

Carrot Seed Oil

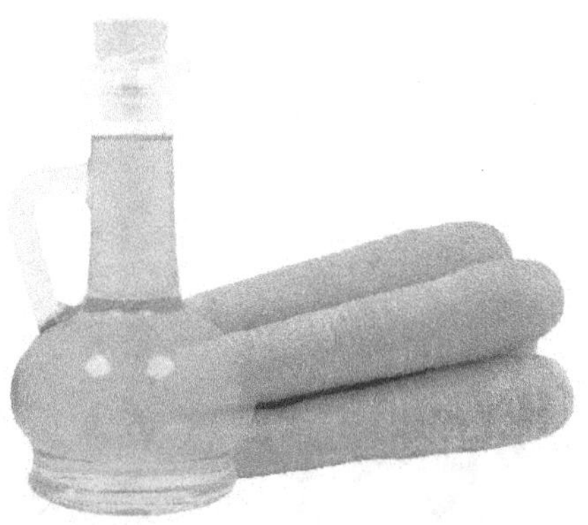

An oil derived from the seed head, Carrot Seed Oil *(Daucus Carota Sativa)* is extraordinarily rich in Vitamin A and has a wonderful warm orange color. One of the richest oils available, carrot see oil is rich in beta carotene and vitamins A & E, and is highly beneficial to hair and skin. Topical application of this oil promotes the formation of new cells and stimulates the production of sebum in dry, scaly skin. Because it is rich in beta-carotene, carrot seed oil is especially beneficial for mature, sensitive, or sun-damaged skin, and for inflammatory skin conditions. Carrot Seed Oil improves the elasticity, tone, and overall appearance of skin. It calms irritated skin while slowing the signs of aging. An excellent oil for eczema, rosacea or psoriasis, this oil offers relief from inflammation, itch, and irritation. Carrot seed oil has antifungal, antibacterial, and anticancer qualities due to its flavonoid content. It is also good for healing scars and lightening dark spots.

Grape Seed Oil

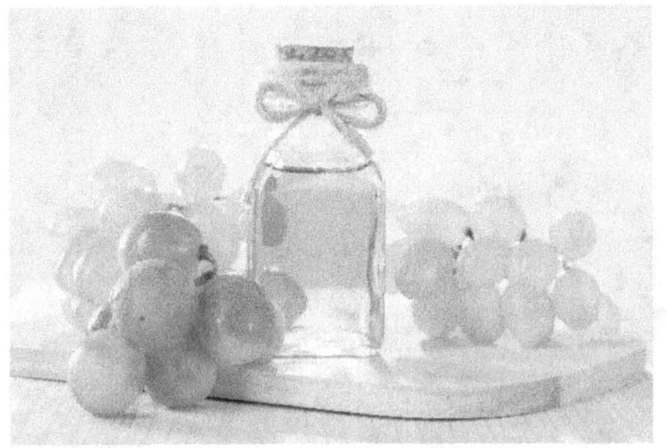

Grape Seed Oil (Vitus vinifera), extracted from the seeds of grapes, is a lightweight oil that easily absorbs into the skin without leaving a greasy feeling. It is extraordinarily rich in linoleic acid (Omega 6), a moisturizing fatty acid quite important for the skin and cell membranes. Grapeseed Oil has been proven to have antimicrobial properties and can be used to treat acne outbreaks. It helps with skin's elasticity and softness as well as retaining moisture. It has a powerful antioxidant called proanthocyanin which helps to even out skin tone when used consistently.

Hazelnut Oil

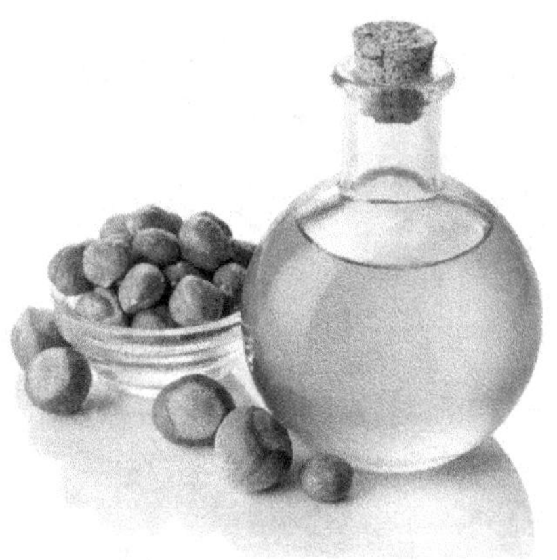

The tree, *Corylus Americana,* native to North America and the *Corylus Avellana* tree, native to Europe give us hazelnuts or filberts. Hazelnut oil must be cold pressed to provide optimal benefits. It contains over 70% oleic and linoleic acids, as well as high amounts of vitamins B and E. The oil itself is considered **mildly astringent** and thus suitable for all skin types. It absorbs quickly and is useful for balancing oily and acne prone skin. Hazelnut oil helps reduce the appearance of pore size. It has anti-aging and moisturizing effects which combat fine lines and wrinkles. It also aids in the regeneration of skin cells. Avoid using Hazelnut oil in formulas intended to deeply moisturize. When used as a single

ingredient, it can draw moisture away from some areas
of the skin leaving dry patches.

Jojoba Oil

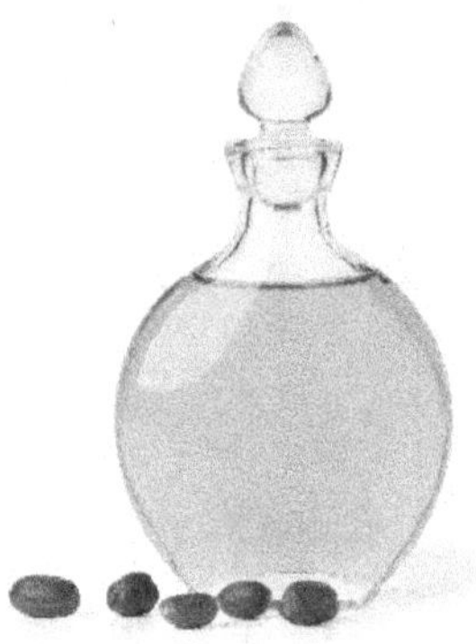

The jojoba plant is a shrub found in southern Arizona, southern California, and northwestern Mexico. It's healing properties have been known to Native Americans for many years. The oil only came into favor in the cosmetic industry in the 1970's. It replaced whale oil which was outlawed in the 1960's as Sperm whales became an endangered species. Previously, whale oil was a major ingredient in cosmetics. Jojoba oil was found to be far superior to whale oil (also known as squalene) with many additional beneficial properties.

The seed of the jojoba plant (Simmondsia chinensis) is about 50% oil by weight. Because it is composed of almost 97% esters of long-chain fatty acids and alcohols, it is a wax by definition. It appears as an oil and so the terms jojoba wax and jojoba oil are used interchangeably. Jojoba is the only plant species known for synthesizing liquid wax. Other plant oils are primarily triglycerides unlike jojoba. As a wax, it has an extremely long shelf life and resistance to oxidation and UV-light degradation.

Jojoba oil is rich in vitamins A, D, and E, tocopherols, and fatty acids. It is easily absorbed and penetrates deeply into the skin. It is naturally antibacterial, antifungal, antiviral, and anti-inflammatory. It is appropriate for any skin type and is hypoallergenic. It works to regenerate skin cells by repairing damage, preventing premature aging, moisturizing, and brightening the skin.

Marula Oil

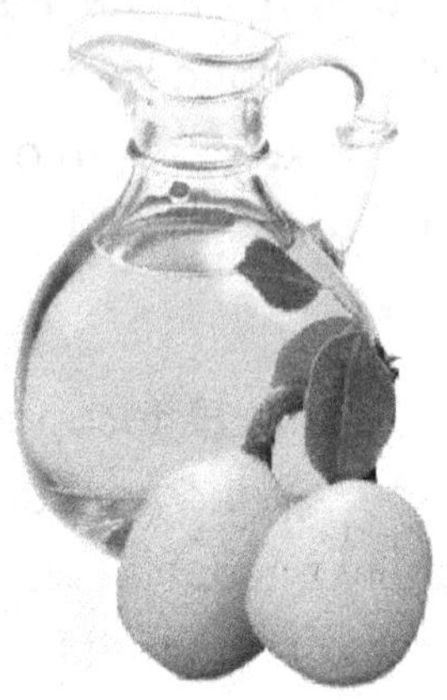

Marula oil is cold/expeller pressed from the kernels found inside the seeds or stones from the fruit of the *Sclerocarya birrea* trees located in several countries in Africa. The oil is composed predominantly of mono-unsaturated fatty acids, oleic acids, phenols, minerals, tocopherols, and protein. It has antimicrobial, anti-inflammatory, and antioxidant properties. The texture of the oil is light and non-greasy which makes it fast absorbing and suitable for all skin types including oily, reactive, and sensitive. The key to Marula's outstanding performance is its fine molecular structure which contributes to its effectiveness as a skin hydrator and protector. It helps heal and reduce acne, blemishes, and scarring, reduces redness, and increases the smoothness of skin. By promoting the production of collagen and elastin, it boosts skin firmness thereby reducing the appearance of fine lines and wrinkles. The antioxidant properties help protect and repair free radical damage from pollution and sun exposure.

Meadowfoam Seed Oil

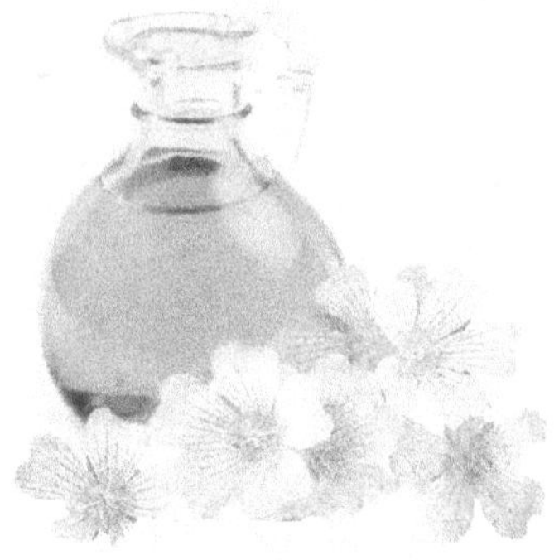

From the wildflower native to northern California, southern Oregon, and Vancouver Island, B.C. meadowfoam *(Limnanthes alba)* seed oil has been studied since the 1950's. The seeds or "nutlets" contain around 30% oil. Meadowfoam seed oil (MSO) is renowned for its unusually high oxidative stability. It is one of the most stable vegetable oils known due to its unique chemical properties. The oil contains over 98% long chain fatty acids and very high-quality triglyceride levels. There are also high euric and eicosenoic acid levels along with the antioxidant vitamins C and E. These properties bestow specific benefits to this oil. In addition to its own oxidative stability, MSO confers that stability to other oils when blended with them. It is highly lubricative and has an enhanced ability to stay on the skin. These benefits are useful in slowing transepidermal water loss (TEWL), preventing dryness and improving the absorption of other nutrients. It moisturizes with a non-greasy feel and also provides UV protection. Because the oil's composition is similar to the body's natural sebum, it helps regulate the oiliness of skin. Its anti-inflammatory properties help acne-prone skin as well. It contains compounds known as glucosinolates which have been found to prevent sun-induced aging by blocking the enzymes which break down collagen.

Moringa Oil

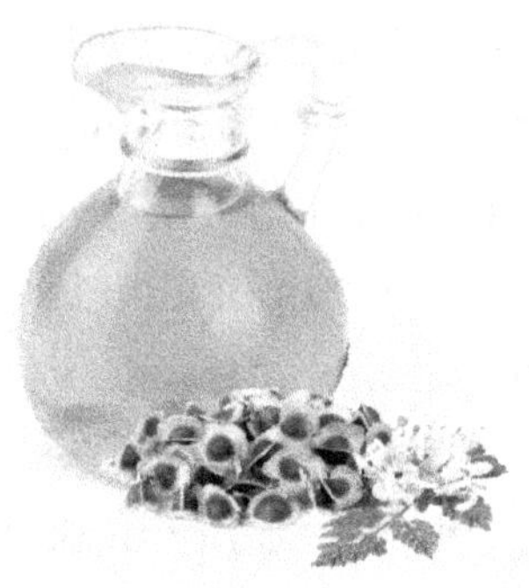

Moringa oleifera (Moringaceae) is a fast-growing softwood tree. It is found in Northern India, the Middle East, and in many African and Asian countries. The rapid growth in these tropical and subtropical climates, even under extreme drought conditions, make it an exceptionally reliable resource. The seeds contain almost 40% oil by weight. Chemical extraction methods can yield close to 100% of the oil, whereas cold pressed methods yield slightly less than 70% of the oil. Moringa oleifera oil (MOO) has been used in folk medicine preparations throughout history. It is rich in Vitamins A, C and E. The tocopherol content is higher than that of other oils. There is a high monounsaturated/saturated fatty acid ratio. More than

70% of the oil is high quality oleic acid. Additional nutrients include behenic acid, a saturated fatty acid that is ideal for many skin care applications. The complete chemical profile for this oil makes it highly resistant to oxidation and gives it strong antioxidant activity. Its topical anti-inflammatory benefits are on par with the medication Dexamethasone. It has an expansive therapeutic profile and a high cosmetic value. MOO cleans dirt from the skin, has anti-bacterial/anti-septic activity, heals insect bites, burns, and cuts, fights black heads, acne, and the negative effects of pollution. One of the many reasons it has received global recognition is because of its anti-aging benefits. Its consistency is similar to sebum which makes it suitable for all skin types. It confers softness and smoothness to dry skin, inhibits free radicals, and gives skin a natural glow.

Pomegranate Seed Oil

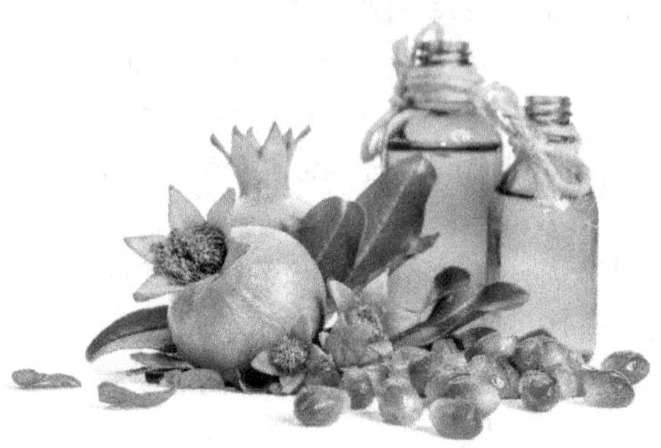

Pomegranate *(Punica granatum)* - a rich, nutritious oil, contains high levels of antioxidants. It helps fight free radicals and skin aging; helps heal, protect, and moisturize dry, cracked, mature, and irritated skin; revitalizes dull or mature skin, assists with wrinkles; improves skin elasticity; and soothes minor skin irritations, including dry skin, eczema, psoriasis, and sunburn. Used topically in skin care, it boosts collagen production and exhibits anti-inflammatory qualities. Its ability to repair skin that is damaged, dry, or aging makes it an ideal ingredient in skin care cosmetics. Pomegranate Oil helps strengthen skin elasticity as well as supporting hormonal balance in both men and women. It is also known for enhancing skin texture. By stimulating cells in the outer layer of skin, Pomegranate

Oil promotes the repair of skin damage by bringing forth a newer layer of skin. Thus, skin appears more youthful. Suitable for all skin types, including oily and acne-prone skin, Pomegranate Oil leaves lasting moisture without leaving a greasy residue or clogging pores.

Pumpkin Seed Oil

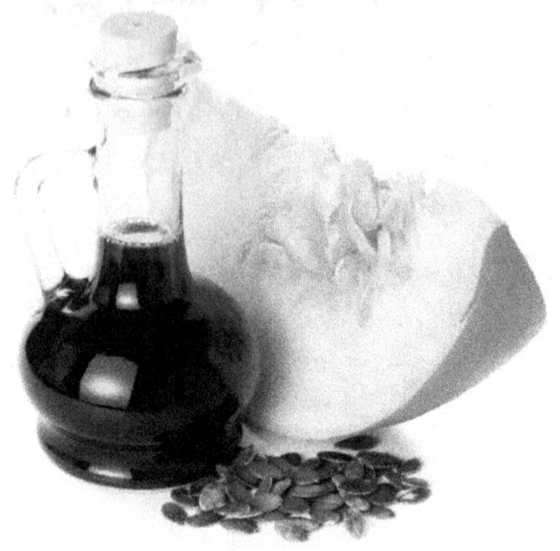

From one of the most recognized fruits on the planet, pumpkin (*Cucurbita pepo* and *Curcurbita maxima)* seed oil is exceptionally rich in vitamins C and E, antioxidants, zinc, and omega 3- and 6- fatty acids. The unique combination of ingredients in pumpkin seed oil (PSO) make it beneficial for cellular regeneration which affects wound healing, premature aging, and skin tone. The balance of omega 3- and 6- fatty acids allow PSO to balance the level of oil in the skin, thereby preventing acne, blackheads, blemishes, and breakouts. The vitamins and minerals help firm and tighten the skin while retaining moisture and providing anti-aging effects. In addition. PSO naturally contains alpha hydroxy acids which facilitate exfoliation and encourage skin cell regeneration.

Rosehip Seed Oil

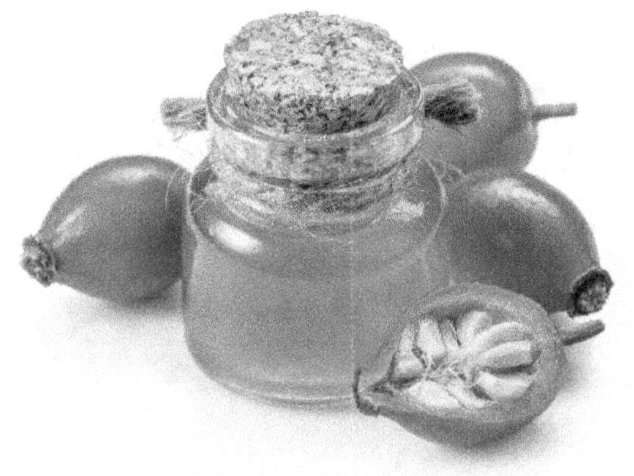

The oil is pressed from the rose hip which is the fruit that grows after the roses have pollinated. The plant, (*Rosa moschata or Rosa rubignosa)* is grown in the southern Andes of Chile. *Rosa Canina*, grown in many areas of South Africa and Europe has also been used. It has properties that are essential for the health of skin. This oil is rich in Vitamin C and essential fatty acids such as linoleic (Omega-6) and linolenic acid (Omega-3). The discovery of this oil has been a game changer in the skin care industry. It is widely used in various skin care products because it is effective in fighting the signs of aging and reducing the problems associated with sun damaged skin. It is a tissue regenerator, and it nourishes and hydrates. It is especially effective with dry skin, cracked skin, stretch marks, age spots, dark spots, burns and scars. The skin nourishing properties help with the healing process.

Sea Buckthorn Berry Oil

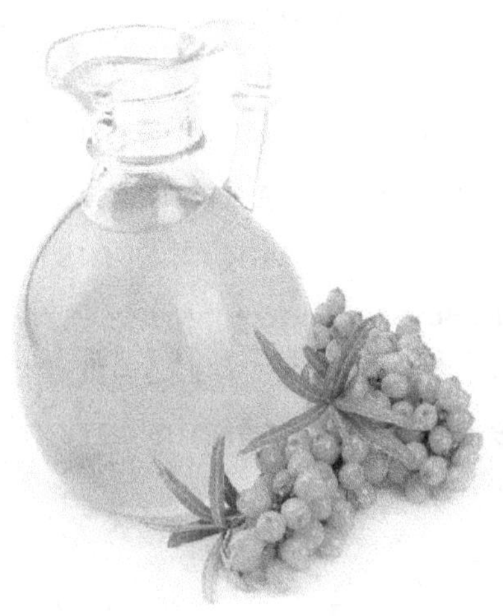

Common sea buckthorn (*Hippophaes rhamnoides)* is a thorny shrub that grows in Europe, Central Asia, Siberia, China, and Tibet. The thorns create difficulties in harvesting the berries which mostly takes place every two years. The oil is taken from the pulp of the berry or the seed and is used in a wide variety of dermatological applications. It is remarkably high in antioxidants (containing 10 times the amount of Vitamin C found in oranges) and boasts copious amounts of phytosterols, Vitamin E, Beta-carotene, and carotenoids. It offers unique and rare unsaturated fatty acids such as palmitoleic acid (omega-7) and gamma-linolenic acid (omega-6). There are close to 200 properties ascribed to this oil. The most significant benefits include skin regeneration and repair, anti-inflammatory, anti-aging, and hydration properties. It improves circulation, facilitates oxygenation of the skin, removes excess toxins, and is easily absorbed into the skin. It protects against infections and prevents allergies. It has a proven track record in the healing of burns, wounds, and restoring skin tissue. It has also been widely used in the treatment of acne, eczema, skin ulcers, cancer, psoriasis, rosacea, and various forms of dermatitis.

Sesame oil

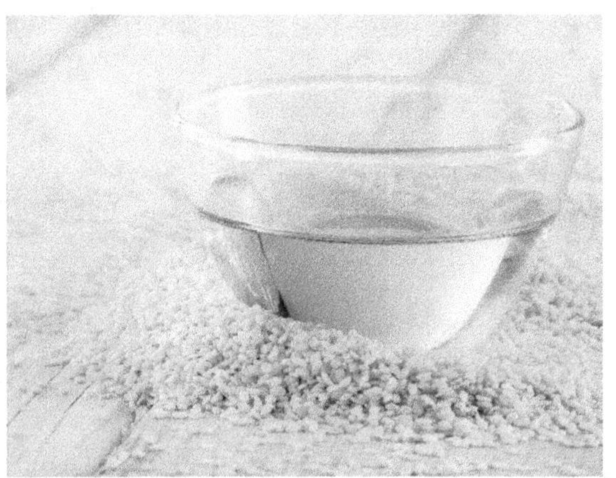

Sesame (*Sesamum indicum*) seeds are approximately 50% oil by weight, taken from an herbaceous plant of many varieties. Believed to have begun in India, it is considered the "Queen of Oilseeds" because it is highly resistant to oxidation giving it a relatively long shelf life. The oil is rich in polyunsaturated fatty acids, especially oleic and linoleic acids. It is also rich in vitamins A, B, and E and many minerals. Unique to sesame oil is the presence of sesamin, sesamolin, sesamol, and related compounds. These are potent antioxidants which contribute to the long shelf life of the oil and provide numerous health benefits to the user. Sesame oil hydrates and nourishes the skin and is absorbed very quickly. It has detoxifying effects beneath the surface of the skin, and it neutralizes free radicals. It is naturally antiviral, antifungal, antibacterial, and anti-inflammatory making it extremely useful in the treatment of acne.

Oil	*Properties*
Argan	Excellent for moisture and anti-aging as well used to fade scars, smooth out the skin's texture, and to treat acne.
Baobab	Restores life back into dull skin.
Black Cumin Seed	Calms inflammation, accelerates healing, helps release and smooth acne scars, smooths skin, leaving it soft and supple.
Carrot Seed	Elasticity and tone. Also calms irritated skin while slowing the signs of aging. Use this oil for eczema and psoriasis. It is good for lightening the skin and lightening dark spots.
Grapeseed	Acne healing, reduces redness, anti-inflammatory, helps with stretch marks and wrinkles.
Hazelnut	Helps minimize pores, tightens and smoothes skin's texture, fights acne by killing bacteria and minimizing both black and whiteheads.
Jojoba	Helps to balance your skin. A non-irritating oil that can be used on all skin types.
Marula	Soothing and healing, reduces the signs of aging as this is loaded with antioxidants. This nutritive oil is soothing for all skin types.
Meadowfoam Seed	Breaks down blackheads and leaves skin soft and smooth. Meadowfoam seed oil is widely used in the beauty industry for its emollient properties and non-greasy feel on the skin.
Moringa	Protect skin from aging with this oil that is rich in antioxidants and highly moisturizing. Will also help reduce redness and inflammation and fight infection.

Pomegranate	Restores the pH balance of your skin while smoothing out fine lines and wrinkles; encourages new cell regeneration to revitalize dull skin. Improves skin elasticity and has healing properties. It's antimicrobial, antibacterial, and anti-inflammatory
Pumpkin Seed	Rich in zinc and selenium, great for fighting acne-causing bacteria. It has a low chance of clogging pores while hydrating and renewing your skin.
Rosehip Seed	High antioxidant content, revitalizes skin and improve texture. Reverses the signs of aging, stretch marks, sun damage, scars, and hyperpigmentation. Use this oil for damaged, dry, mature, and irritated skin.
Seabuckthor n Seed	Ant-inflammatory oil. Helps imbalances in your body from the inside out. Reduces redness and regenerates your skin cells. Slows signs of aging, protects against the sun, and increases healthy skin structure.
Sesame	Promotes wound healing as well as kills acne causing bacteria. This oil has tremendous antibacterial qualities. Can be used as a protectant against the sun. Helps with the texture and appearance of your skin.

Chapter 5

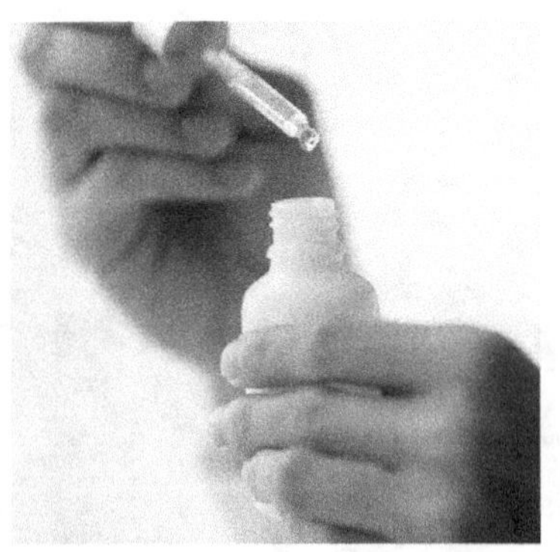

Creating Your Own
Perfect Facial Oil

Because all these oils are multifunctional, you will notice many oils in several categories. Experience and time-tested results have guided the creation of these particular formulas. However, armed with information, you may also use your own inner wisdom to create your perfect facial oil blend.

Top 6 Areas of Concern
(Oil Cheat Sheet)

Concerns	Oils
Aging, Wrinkles, Crows Feet, Sagging Skin	Argan Pomegranate Rosehip Marula Jojoba
Dry Skin, Dullness, Dry Patches	Marula Pumpkin Seed Moringa Meadowfoam Seed
Inflammation, Redness Eczema, Rosacea, Psoriasis	Black Cumin Carrot Moringa Sea Buckthorn
Oily Skin, Acne, Breakouts, Pore Minimizing	Hazelnut Jojoba Grapeseed
Prevention, General wellbeing and Maintenance	Baobab Moringa Argan Sea Buckthorn
Uneven skin texture, Scarring, Dark Spots	Rosehip Sea Buckthorn Sesame Argan

Chapter 6

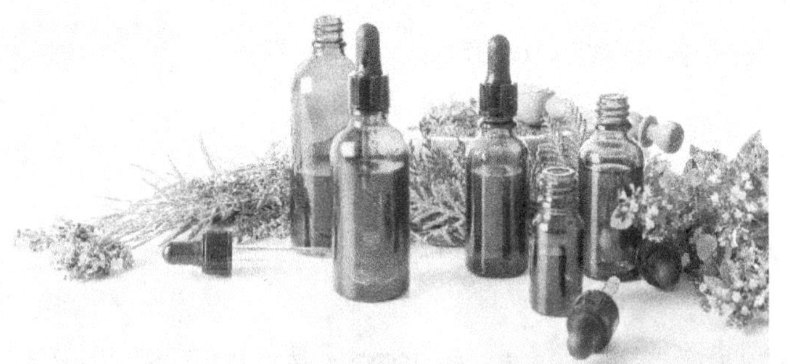

Effective Skin Care Formulas

The formulas presented are elegantly simple. The chief objective is to create the most effective, targeted, formula with the simplest ingredients. All formulas are a total weight of 1oz. All necessary items can be purchased through Amazon.com. We do not get any commission from your purchase.

What you will need

- 1oz Amber Bottle(s) with droppers for finished product

- Plant Oils – you won't need more than 2oz of each oil. Each oil must be the only ingredient and not part of an oil blend. More than 2 oz of oil will probably not be used before it expires. Check for the expiration date and lot # on each purchase. Expired oils will not give you the results you want. Most oils are good for at least one year from the date they are packaged. If the oils are expired or nearing their expiration date, they can be returned and/or exchanged. Lot numbers are only important in case of a product recall.

- Small kitchen scale - These should measure in tenths of ounces and have a "tare" function which is discussed below.

- Clean space to work away from direct sunlight.

Directions

1. Make sure the scale is calibrated to zero.
2. Weigh a plain amber bottle without the dropper by placing it on the scale.
3. If your scale will allow you to reset the weight at zero (tare) with the amber bottle in place, do so. If not, write down the weight of the bottle so that it can be subtracted from the total weight of the formula in the end.
4. Slowly pour, or use your dropper to place ingredients into the bottle on the scale to achieve the desired amounts - 0.2, 0.3, or 0.5 oz. Using the dropper to slowly add the desired amount of oil is a better option for beginners.
5. Once all ingredients have been added, close the bottle, and shake well.

6. Keep oils in a cool place away from direct sunlight.
7. Label and date the oil for future reference.
8. Oils should be effective for a minimum of 1 year.

Whether you use one of the formulas below or create one of your own, it's important that you follow the formulating rules. The oil that addresses your main objective must be at least 50% of the facial oil formula. If it is less, your results will not be the same. If you only choose 2 oils for your formula 50/50 is a good bet. A formula which is 75% of your targeted oil will also work. When formulas require more substantial therapeutic effects, we recommend using 3 oils. This is the case when addressing complicated skin conditions. Here, there are multiple areas of concern which create the skin conditions. Using more than 3 oils can create formulating concerns, possibly decreasing the effectiveness of the oil blend. Even in formulas containing 3 oils, the ingredient delivering your main goal should be at least 50% of the formula. It is easier to split the second half of the 50% between the remaining two oils. To ensure success, the remaining 2 oils should be from the same category.

Effective Formulas

Anti- Aging Facial Oil #1

Argan	0.5oz
Marula	0.3oz
Rosehip Seed	0.2oz

Anti-Aging Facial Oil #2

Pomegranate	0.5oz
Argan	0.3oz
Jojoba	0.2oz

Daily Maintenance/Natural Glow Facial Oil #1

Marula	0.5oz
Moringa	0.5oz

Daily Maintenance/Natural Glow Facial Oil #2

Pumpkin	0.5oz
Meadowfoam	0.5oz

Dry/Dull Skin Facial Oil #1
      Moringa   0.5oz
      Pumpkin   0.5oz

Dry/Dull Skin Facial Oil #2
      Meadowfoam 0.5oz
      Sesame   0.5oz

Eczema Facial Oil #1
      Jojoba   0.5oz
      Seabuckthorn 0.3oz
      Black Cumin   0.2oz

Eczema Facial Oil #2
      Moringa   0.5oz
      Seabuckthorn 0.3oz
      Carrot   0.2oz

Oily/Acne Skin Facial Oil #1
      Hazelnut   0.5oz
      Jojoba   0.3oz

                Grapeseed   0.2oz

Oily/Acne Skin Facial Oil #2
        Hazelnut   0.7oz
        Grapeseed   0.3oz

Rosacea Facial Oil #1
        Seabuckthorn 0.4oz
        Black Cumin   0.4oz
        Jojoba   0.2oz

Rosacea Facial Oil #2
        Rosehip Seed 0.4oz
        Moringa   0.4oz
        Jojoba   0.2oz

Scar Fade Facial Oil #1
        Seabuckthorn 0.5oz
        Argan   0.5oz

Scar Fade Facial Oil #2
        Rosehip Seed 0.5oz
        Seabuckthorn 0.5oz

Your Facial Oil
Worksheet

Because it is not possible to get every desirable property into one formula, it is important to prioritize the results you are looking for. To that end, we have listed the top areas of concern below. Please choose the number 1, 2, and possibly 3 areas of concern. This will help you to choose the oils that will most benefit what you.

What is the Main Area of Concern?

____

Anti-Aging	Wrinkle	Uneven tone/dark spots
Sagging Skin	Tough/rough skin	Dull/Dry skin
Large Pores	Acne	Oiliness
Scars	Prevention	Redness/ Inflammation

What is the Second Area of Concern?

____

Anti-Aging	Wrinkles	Uneven tone/dark spots
Sagging Skin	Tough/rough skin	Dull/Dry skin
Large Pores	Acne	Oiliness
Scars	Prevention	Redness/ Inflammation

Based on what you have chosen, check the "Oil Cheat Sheet" for the oil(s) that will best meet your needs.

If you have only one concern, choose an oil that fits that need.

1 concern - use 100% of the oils from that category.

2 concerns – 75% of oil from category#1 and 25% of oil from category #2

3 concerns – 50% of oil from category #1, 25% of oil from category #2, and 25% of oil from category #3.

As you can see, many oils can address more than one area of concern. For example, the two concerns of dry skin and anti-aging could be addressed with Marula oil alone. However, the addition of another oil from either dry skin or anti-aging category would boost the effectiveness overall.

Chapter 7

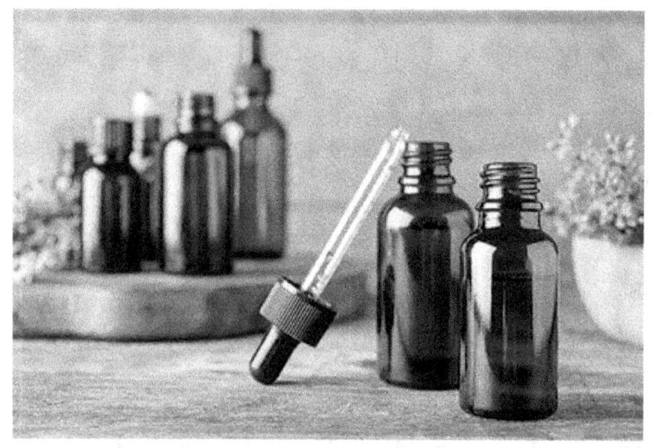

Helpful Tips

Chapter 7

Helpful Tips

It is important to remember that all these oils are powerful and will effect change with constant use. If not daily, they should be applied at least 4 times a week to be effective.

There are some oils that you shouldn't mix because they will be serving cross purposes. For instance, Hazelnut oil will definitely help to minimize oiliness. It should not be mixed with oils used for moisturization.

If you have several concerns, for example, dry skin, wrinkles, scars, and rosacea, you should select your top two concerns to start. Using oils for scar repair or inflamed skin will get you results, but will not reduce the appearance or wrinkles as quickly as if you were using oils in that category.

Trying to mix oils to address several concerns at once will lead to disappointment. In general, the concentration and efficacy of any one oil will be

reduced (diluted) by the presence of oils with other properties.

If you are suffering from inflamed skin due to Rosacea, Eczema or Psoriasis, the oils that address these concerns can be applied at any time. In this case, they can be applied as needed to reduce inflammation and provide relief from symptoms.

It is important to seek medical attention for any serious concerns.

Conclusion

Now you know. The wonderful field of facial oils is full of discovery. It is old and new at the same time. Some oils have been used for centuries; others are still being discovered. There are scientific studies that show this is not a field of dreams and hyperbole. There are significant benefits to using facial oils which can be helpful for everyone.

Facial oils are beneficial for hydrating, moisturizing, protecting, healing, and enhancing. Simple, single oils have unique therapeutic benefits from acne to anti-aging. Facial oil blends take advantage of multi functioning ingredients and proven therapeutic formulations to enhance and increase the benefits of the individual oils.

You now have all the basic information you need to create an effective facial oil, to include them in your daily regimen, and to increase the qualities you want most.

After researching and writing this book for consumers, it became clear that at least one commercially available facial oil should be recommended. At some point, a formulator may just want to purchase a product. There are many companies and products from which to choose. However, it was simply not possible to evaluate every facial oil product, notwithstanding the ethics of other companies.

Bibliography

The Enigma of Bioactivity and Toxicity of Botanical Oils for Skin Care [5]

Skin hydration in postmenopausal women: argan oil benefit with oral and/or topical use

https://www.ncbi.nlm.nih.gov/pmc/articles/PMC5796020/(woundhealing,anti-inflammatoryeffectsofskinoilsingeneral)

Abundance of active ingredients in sea-buckthorn oil

T3*Nigella sativa* L. (Black Cumin): A Promising Natural Remedy for Wide Range of Illnesses

Review Dermatological effects of Nigella sativa

Anti-Inflammatory and Skin Barrier Repair Effects of Topical Application of Some Plant Oils

African seed oils of commercial importance — Cosmetic applications

(Zielińska and Nowak, 2014)Beauty in Baobab: a pilot study of the safety and efficacy of *Adansonia digitata* seed oil

Value addition in sesame: A perspective on bioactive components for enhancing utility and profitability

SESAME OIL https://www.agmrc.org/commodities-products/grains-oilseeds/meadowfoam

https://plantbreeding.oregonstate.edu/plantbreeding/research/meadowfoam-breeding-program

"https://al-bab.com/argan-tree-life

Nutraceutical potentialities of Tunisian Argan oil based on its physicochemical properties and fatty acid content as assessed through Bayesian network analyses .

The effect of dietary and/or cosmetic argan oil on postmenopausal skin elasticity

Jojoba oil - Wikipedia.

Solidification of oil liquids by encapsulation within porous hollow silica microspheres of narrow size distribution for pharmaceutical and cosmetic applications

[20]Acute Effects of Transdermal Administration of Jojoba Oil on Lipid Metabolism in Mice

Acute Effects of Transdermal Administration of Jojoba Oil on Lipid Metabolism in Mice

Moringa oleifera Seeds and Oil: Characteristics and Uses for Human Health

In vitro anti-allergic activity of Moringa oleifera Lam. extracts and their isolated compounds

Expanding the anti-inflammatory potential of Moringa oleifera: topical effect of seed oil on skin inflammation and hyperproliferation

Organic Moringa Oil

Promising features of Moringa oleifera oil: recent updates and perspectives

Moringa oleifera Leaf Extracts as Multifunctional Ingredients for "Natural and Organic" Sunscreens and Photoprotective Preparations

www.ingramcontent.com/pod-product-compliance
Lightning Source LLC
Chambersburg PA
CBHW070944250726
48663CB00001B/59